Inside-Out Weight Loss

Change your relationship with food forever with
NLP and Hypnotherapy

Louise Dorrian

British Library Cataloguing in Publication Data.

A catalogue record for this book is available from the British Library.

ISBNs Paperback 9781780921891
ePub 9781780921907
PDF 9781780921914

MX Publishing, 335 Princess Park Manor, Royal Drive, London, N11 3GX.
www.mxpublishing.co.uk
Cover Design by www.staunch.com

Contents

Inside – Out Weight Loss

Introduction

Welcome to a transformational approach to weight loss. It's simple really – the reason you have tried to lose weight before and not been successful is because you have been doing it the wrong way! Losing weight successfully is about changing your relationship with food, learning to appreciate yourself, doing the best for yourself and creating a healthier future.

Eating plans, diets, weight loss clubs, counting calories or points, slimming pills and meal replacements are all things you do from the outside when the issue lies on the *inside*. I fully advocate healthy eating and exercise but unless you have tackled the reasons why you are overweight in the first place and what is keeping you overweight, then you are wasting your time, effort and probably a lot of money as well on the 'external' stuff.

You might have also noticed that engaging in all the 'external' stuff you are handing over control to something or someone else – the 'diets', the weight loss club leader, the scientists who develop the pills etc. and putting your faith and hope in them. You will most probably have felt let down by them too (or blame them for your failure) but at the same time knowing deep down inside that it's no-one else's responsibility but your own. 'Inside – Out' puts you back in charge in a way that means you can easily control your relationship with food and the associated behaviours and feelings. That way, you lose weight and keep it off permanently.

So, by engaging in and following the Inside-Out Weight Loss approach you will **lose as much weight as you want** as a result of taking control, resolving the issues that make you over eat, enjoying the responsibility and freedom in creating the lifestyle you want, and strange as it may seem to you at the moment - you will learn to really *love food.*

Some of the slimmest, healthiest people I know have a passion for food and enjoy cooking, eating out and socialising around food. So you can let go of that perception right now that to be slim you have to deny yourself tasty food and eat only tiny portions – it's just not true.

Inside-Out Weight Loss works by changing the way your mind works. That might sound a bit dramatic but if you think about anyone who had turned their life around, perhaps by over coming a disability, conquering a fear or achieving something no-one considered possible, you will come to the conclusion that the biggest change these people made was in their head. How they thought, which changed how they felt, which resulted in their changed behaviour. And ALL changes to long-term behaviour are made unconsciously through 're-programming' your unconscious mind. Deciding consciously to only eat calorie restricted ready meals every night for dinner won't work for weight loss long term because your relationship with food will not have changed unconsciously. That's not to say that certain types of behaviour won't *contribute* to your weight loss – I'm presuming that you consciously decided to pick up this book and read it and that you will consciously decide to listen to the recordings that accompany it. Some of the 'actions' and suggestions in the book require you to consciously monitor what and how you eat or to consciously plan activity into your day. The underlying thoughts and patterns that enable you to *sustain* this control and patterns of behaviour are however made at an unconscious level. The changes that result in long term behavioural shifts happen unconsciously by 're-programming' the way you think. We are only able to hold 7 (plus or minus 2) items in our minds consciously - everything else is unconscious. Which is probably just as well or else it would take forever to do anything and can you imagine giving *everything* your full attention all the time? It would be exhausting and confusing! Inside-Out Weight Loss shows you how and guides you towards making changes in your unconscious mind so that your behaviour changes without you even having to think about it consciously.

Incorporating NLP (Neuro-Linguistic Programming) and Hypnotherapy, Inside-Out Weight Loss is an effective, safe and easy way to lose weight. You can find out more about NLP and Hypnotherapy in the Appendix.

Structure

This book takes you through a program of actions to firstly resolve compulsive and habitual dependence on food and other psychological drivers to over eat, and then it focuses on making healthy choices and allowing activity into your lifestyle. Each of the 3 parts is supported by a hypnotic recording on the Inside-Out website and you will be directed on how to access these recordings at the appropriate section in the book.

'On the Inside', 'Taking Control' and 'Making it Last' form part one and this guides you gently through the process of making behavioural changes that will last for a lifetime. We start on the inside resolving issues that you might not even be aware of but that impact on your behaviour and what you choose to eat on a daily basis. When people are happy, contented and in control of their behaviour they don't over-eat. People that over-eat do so because it fulfils some other purpose than to alleviate physical hunger.

We then move on to what I call getting you 'comfortably in control' of your eating habits. Even after resolving issues that made you over-eat in the first place, your body and mind is so used to you eating for other reasons that it needs to be 're-programmed' to what is essentially the normal pattern of behaviour. You will become more tuned into the 'act of eating'.

We will look at *how* you are approaching the whole change to your outlook, habits and routines. We are creating a future that includes you at your ideal weight so this stage will ensure that you have the best possible foundations to build on. Making the changes on the inside that allow you to replace unhelpful attitudes and thoughts with positive, powerful ones, makes it possible to succeed in what you never considered to be achievable.

Part 2 supports you in making healthy, balanced food choices for a healthy lifestyle, to complement the changes you have already made. You probably want to imagine that when you are slim you are also healthy and full of energy so you can really enjoy becoming the you that you always dreamed of – therefore what you eat is important. Like I said in the introduction this program is about letting *you* enjoy the responsibility and control of making the changes and decisions that will result in you losing weight and keeping it off forever. So there are no diets or meal plans, no one to tell you what you 'should' or 'shouldn't' eat. At this point you will already have made huge changes to how you think about food, and the habits you had around food. You will already be finding yourself making healthier choices and loving food for what it is: just that- 'food' – not an emotional crutch, friend, diversion or hobby.

Here, we are moving forward to recognising food as a source of nutrition to make you feel and look great. There is no jargon or boring, long winded explanation about the chemical or biological composition of food just a common sense guide to balancing what you eat to gain maximum nutritional value from it. You will also learn how to deal with the cravings we all get from time to time!

The third and final part coaches you to integrate more activity into your life – supporting the healthy lifestyle you are already adopting. Everyone knows that keeping active is vital to good health. There are plenty of thin people out there who aren't fit and you can usually tell just by looking at them – they don't look good! The thin people that look good, feel good and have loads of energy are the ones who have exercise as part of their normal routine along with healthy eating habits. Here the program will guide you to keep active and make it a part of *your* routine, give you the motivation to get on with it and make it something you really enjoy doing.

How Inside-Out Weight Loss Works

To begin with it's useful to understand why what you have done in the past to lose weight didn't work, or didn't work for long.

The universally accepted formula for losing weight is:

Energy in (i.e. calories from food and drink) < Energy out.

I am sure that if you have tried to lose weight before or have any idea about how your body works then you will agree with that formula. This is absolutely correct – I agree with it too! However, that would be the answer if we were working with laboratory rats, but if you are reading this I am quite sure that you are most likely human. Diets, meal plans and meal replacements follow this formula but also give rise to another (completely unscientific) equation of my own:

Purposely restricting energy in = irritability, misery, hunger and obsession with food.

Have you ever wondered why some humans struggle to control their weight yet you never see a wild animal that is overweight? The only animals that you will see that are overweight are the ones that have been over fed by the humans that feed them. The reason is that animals eat for one reason only – to live. They take in enough energy to balance with the energy they need to live. This is also true for human babies − you won't remember consciously but when you were a baby you demanded food when you were hungry and stopped when your hunger was satisfied.

The problems start when we humans start to develop a 'relationship' with food. Food is no longer just about our instinct to survive, it starts to hold so many more meanings and purposes for us. In terms of what food means − it can be highly symbolic, for example in some cultures, being used as offerings to gods, in religious festivals, celebrations, to show wealth or generosity, to show love, friendship or compassion. Withholding food can be used to demonstrate power, to punish or show displeasure. It therefore follows that how we receive food will also carry meaning − what, how, when and how much we eat can be taken to show respect/disrespect, trust, love, conformity and obedience.

This 'relationship' starts to sound very complex and tricky to manage, but when you add in the psychological attachment and habitual dependence on food as well it seems like a nightmare!

Just like all the things you do often enough, your eating habits become ingrained in your unconscious mind. And like other unconscious behaviours they are very difficult to change consciously − just try to consciously 'unlearn' to ride a bike or tie your shoe laces!

Your complex behaviours around food need to be tackled at an unconscious level to have any lasting impact on your relationship with it.

So why would the diet industry treat us like animals and ignore our complex relationship with food as *the most significant* reason people become overweight?

Well, firstly, because the diet industry makes millions of pounds and dollars from people who are compulsive dieters who fail and come back time and time again to buy their products, and secondly because they don't understand how our conscious and unconscious minds work together to form our eating behaviours.

Luckily, I *do* understand that what lies in your unconscious mind forms the basis of an unhelpful relationship with food. By tackling the issues at an unconscious level to complement what you do consciously, losing weight will become a natural, easy and rewarding process of change.

So you can stop wasting your time and money on diets that make you feel miserable, remove any enjoyment from food and leave you feeling hungry. You can embark on a process of almost effortless change that will mean you rapidly reach your ideal weight and start living a healthy lifestyle.

Inside-Out Weight Loss works by firstly giving you the tools that allow you to become aware of your eating habits. You will be able to identify compulsive eating patterns and habitual behaviour and become more in control of why you eat. You will distinguish between emotional and physical hunger and break the unconscious connection that drives you to over-eat. You will further change your relationship with food by 're-programming' your eating habits and reaching a comfortable level of control. This level of awareness and control is achieved through a combination of conscious and unconscious change. Consciously you will use some simple techniques and tools to learn new ways of relating to food. By listening to the recordings regularly you will make significant changes at an unconscious level – without even realising it.

I am guessing that the way you currently relate to food and the part it plays in your life is something quite central to you and your lifestyle. Most overweight people have an overwhelming connection to food that features prominently in their waking hours. Changing that will obviously mean changes to lifestyle, thoughts, feelings, relationships with others and daily routines. It is therefore really important that how you approach your weight loss transformation complements and supports your future outcomes. To 'make it last' you will gain techniques to create the lifestyle you want and deal with the challenges on the way.

Each part of the book gives you 'Actions' to complete, there are 16 in total. Read the Actions through first a couple of times as some of them require you to have your eyes closed so it's best to be clear on what you are doing first. Carrying out all of the Actions will result in you changing your relationship with food forever and reaching your ideal weight, so be sure to do them all and listen to the recordings when you are directed to do so.

It's great that you have decided that now is the time to finally lose the weight you want to and gain the healthy, slim enjoyable lifestyle you always thought out of your reach. By adopting the Inside-Out Weight Loss approach you WILL succeed. You can take as much time as you need to go through the exercises and listen to the recordings. Some people complete the book and actions in just a few weeks, and you will start noticing changes from week one.

Case Study

Farquhar, a project manager in the construction industry struggled with his weight for many years and despite joining weight loss clubs and dieting still couldn't lose the weight that was beginning to seriously affect his health. This is what he says: *"The Inside-Out Weight Loss program has changed my whole outlook on and attitude towards food. I no longer feel the need to eat to a schedule or eat all the food on my plate. I am quite happy eating smaller portions and eating only when I am hungry. The program has given me a more positive mental attitude and I feel a lot more confident about myself, my body and the way I look.*

I find that listening to the audio recordings last thing at night is extremely relaxing and helps me get a full nights restful sleep, but listening to the recording in the morning, before I go to work, I feel invigorated and confident for the rest of the day.

Over a four week period, which covered 2 weeks family holiday, summer barbecues and a week of extended working hours I was able to lose 8lbs with very little effort on my behalf.

The program is simple to follow and the techniques are easy to apply during your day. I felt the benefits within the first few days and am now showing the benefits after just a few weeks.

For me the program works not only for weight loss but for an overall improvement of personal attitude and confidence".

Part One

On The Inside

We'll start by dealing with the reasons behind why you over-eat and struggle to lose weight. When you become aware of situations, habits and compulsions that lead to over-eating you can start to make changes to alter those behaviours forever.

As with any process of change it's a really good idea to keep a record of your progress along with any concerns, achievements and general observations. Writing things down helps to rationalise thoughts and provides a visual record of just how well you are doing! Therefore I recommend that you keep an 'Inside-Out' journal and note down your thoughts, progress and challenges daily. In conjunction with this and to track and become aware of your eating patterns you are also going to complete a 'food-mood' diary:

17

Your Food-Mood Diary

Action!   *1: Food-Mood Diary*

For the next few weeks complete a 'Food-Mood' diary in your journal. This should look something like the table on the next page – which you can recreate in your journal or keep a copy on your computer. A downloadable copy is available on the website: www.insideoutweightloss.com/resources-and-downloads

Be honest about what you record in your Food-Mood diary – no one else needs to see it so you may as well put down *everything* that you eat and be interested to see if a pattern emerges.

As you get used to stopping and thinking about how you feel when you eat something you will start to notice that some of your 'hunger' is not physical but emotional or habitual.

Food/Mood Diary

	Food/Drink	Mood (what were you feeling like at the time e.g. angry, upset, happy, bored, stressed etc, or neutral)
Breakfast time		
Morning		
Lunch time		
Afternoon		
Dinner time		
Evening		

19

Emotional and habitual eating

Over time you may have become conditioned to eat when you feel sad, angry, depressed or hurt. It's not necessary to examine the personal historical reason for this but it may have been connected to a stimulus/response situation such as food being given when you were upset as a child. As a result you may have started to view food as a comfort – something to 'take the pain away'. Perhaps you have used food as a diversion from other issues in your life, it makes you feel better while you are eating it, but you feel worse when you stop and realise how much you have eaten – so you eat more to feel better again. It's a horrible vicious circle. Often you will look for the temporary 'high' that comes from sugary foods – which will boost your blood sugar levels making you feel better but then your blood sugar levels will crash very quickly afterwards making you feel even worse.

Our brains are wired to maintain a level of endorphins that makes us feel good. When these levels are depleted because of stress or anxiety we often crave something that will give us a 'boost' (literally something that will boost our endorphin levels). A really quick way to do this is to eat something fatty or sugary – but of course we know that isn't good for us so we experience a short relief from the unpleasant feelings inside but know we are doing ourselves harm in the long term – and this makes us feel bad again!

behaviour that may emerge from your Mood diary is 'habitual' compulsive eating. This is where you feel the compulsion to eat because perhaps you are bored or because you always eat when you watch TV or go to the cinema for example. Other eating behaviours which fall into this category are – finishing off your children's leftovers, finishing all the food on your plate, eating whatever is given to you in case you offend your host, always having a biscuit or cake with a cup of tea or coffee. These are habits and simply becoming more aware of them by recording them in your food-mood diary may make you think twice about doing it, but often habits are difficult to break consciously, without a new strategy.

So, by keeping a record of your eating behaviour you will start to see that you eat for 3 reasons:

1. Because you are physically hungry
2. Because you are 'emotionally' hungry – compulsive eating
3. Because you have learned unhelpful food habits – habitual eating

Case study
Sam who is a busy mother and works with special needs children found the Inside-Out program really easy to follow and quickly differentiated her physical from emotional hunger; she says it was *"like a light being switched on – I have changed my relationship with food forever"*. She lost 9lbs and dropped a dress size in only 5 weeks.

Action! 2: Emotional and Habitual Eating

It's reasons 2 and 3 that are keeping you overweight. Go back to your Food-Mood diary and mark down the numbers 1, 2 or 3 next to the entries to indicate the reason for eating against the food you ate.

You are now taking a very powerful position – becoming witness to your own behaviour. By taking a step outside of yourself and observing what you do, you can identify behaviours that you weren't aware of before. That puts you in the ideal position to change them!

You can identify patterns from your food/mood diary of when you eat 'emotionally' and 'habitually' and you can now recognise situations that may lead to these types of eating behaviour. In your journal - write down these situations or stimuli. For example:

Emotional eating -

"I eat when I feel [emotion or feeling]",

"I feel [emotion or feeling] because [circumstances, memory, stimulus]"

For example: *"I eat when I feel <u>anxious</u>",*

"I feel <u>anxious</u> because <u>my boss sets me unreasonable targets</u>"*

cont./

Habitual eating -

"I eat when [situation]"

"The reason why I eat in this situation is..."

For example: *"I eat <u>when I clear away the kids' leftovers</u>"*

> *"The reason why I eat in this situation is that <u>I don't like to waste food</u>"**

*It's not absolutely necessary for you to consciously know why you have compulsive behaviour – the reasons will be held in your unconscious mind. Listening to the recording and practising your own focused thinking (which you are guided through later in the chapter) will access and resolve these issues.

Your inner voice

So you have now identified the times, places and situations where you over-eat and will be more aware of the factors contributing to that behaviour. We all have 'strategies' for everything that we do whether it is how we get ready for work or our day ahead, how we organise our shopping trips or spend our leisure time. Strategies involve following a pattern of behaviour in response to particular stimuli or triggers. But the good thing is that you can change your strategies by 're-programming' how you respond to triggers and installing new strategies. But before you do that, go back to your 'witness position' and this time think about how you talk to yourself. Take a moment to think about what sort of things your internal voice is saying to you, right now and when you feel compelled to over-eat or after you have eaten something you consider to be 'bad'. More than likely, its not very complimentary. Perhaps you berate yourself for eating something you decide you 'shouldn't have', or maybe you call yourself names or tell yourself that you are disgusted with your behaviour or decide what other people think of you and tell yourself that too. Imagine how you would feel if other people talked to you the way you talk to yourself. Imagine saying those things to someone you love – how does it make you feel? Not good I bet. But constantly disappointing yourself can lead to self-loathing and that constant internal fight between denial and reward, seeking comfort and then berating yourself is stressful, not to mention mentally exhausting. Stop verbally abusing yourself. You wouldn't put up with it from anybody else so change that internal voice into one that is supporting, loving and kind – you deserve it. Praise yourself for having taken the first steps towards changing your lifestyle forever and appreciate all the good things that you do for yourself and others.

Action!   ***3: Your Kind Inner Voice***

Write a list in your journal now of all the positive things about yourself (there are plenty of them) for example: "I am a good friend and always have time to listen" or "I have patience with my kids" or "I take good care of my pets" ***and*** *"I am a good person".*

Acknowledge all the good things you are and do and then acknowledge the fact that you recognise that you need to make changes to your relationship with food, and that you are working towards a new healthier lifestyle. Allow your internal voice to practise patience and understanding when you feel you have gone off track – in the same way you would if a child made a mistake or got confused. Your internal voice can be encouraging and supportive – after all it's a part of you, and all parts of you have your best interests at heart.

New strategy generator

As I said earlier, our brains are designed to work with strategies – our actions are a sequence of events constructed around our thoughts, feelings and information we take in from the outside world through our senses. Compulsive and habitual eating patterns of behaviour are also 'strategic' – there is a trigger and then a sequence of internal events that result in you achieving a result. The trigger could be an emotion or event resulting in a familiar internal dialogue, recalled internal feeling, sound and/or image. This leads you to take a particular action (e.g. eating a huge slice of chocolate cake when you feel upset or eating a bucket of popcorn every time you go to the cinema) to complete the strategy and achieve a result (e.g. to provide comfort or fulfil a pattern of behaviour).

But you can **make new strategies**. The most effective way to do this is by changing them on both your conscious and unconscious levels. On a conscious level you can use the exercise on the next page to target specific triggers and change the way you respond. This exercise is particularly good for habitual eating patterns (strategies). It works with the way your mind forms a strategy through its representation of images, sounds and feelings and enables you to re-program and form new connections with a new behaviour in response to a trigger situation. Once these patterns are in place they become unconscious.

Action!   4: New Strategy Generator

Think about a situation where you want to respond differently

1. **Look downward to your left** and talk to yourself internally – asking yourself *"what do I want to do differently in this situation"* and *"what would I look like, what would I hear and see in this new way of behaving"*?

2. **Look upwards to your right** and visualise yourself carrying out this new behaviour exactly as you want it to be. (If you have difficulty seeing yourself behaving in this new way, you can think of someone else who already does it.) Watch your new behaviour as if you are seeing yourself in a movie. Make all the changes you need to make to what you see and hear until you have it exactly as you want it. Notice how other people react to you in this movie and what they see and hear too.

3. **Look downward to your right** and feel yourself stepping into that movie now – as if you are actually there looking out from your own eyes. See what you can see, what you can hear and notice how that makes you **feel**.

4. Check that everything feels right and go through the process from 3 again and make any changes you want to make. Do it twice more.

5. Think about the stimulus or trigger that will be your prompt for this new behaviour and imagine that happening in the future. Imagine yourself acting in this new way and feel how good it feels to have that response.

    You might need to practise this a few times and once you have the routine right – try getting yourself into a really relaxed, comfortable state and closing your eyes before carrying out the steps.

Focused thinking and hypnosis

Changing your strategies at an unconscious level is something you can do yourself effectively through focused thinking and listening to the Inside-Out Weight Loss hypnotic recordings. Focused thinking is also known as Self-Hypnosis.

Often patterns of behaviour resulting in compulsive or emotional eating have their origins deep in your unconscious mind. You might not even be aware of the event or situation that formed the initial connection between eating and feeling different. A lot of our behaviours as adults stem from how we experienced events, emotions and relationships in our past, sometimes originating in early childhood. At that stage, connections were formed between triggers and responses – with the intention of putting us in the best and happiest position. Those responses may have been useful at the time but might not serve us as well now. For example you might have been encouraged to 'eat everything on your plate' and you did because it made your mother happy, and that felt good. However eating everything on your plate now really only makes you overweight – especially if there is too much on your plate to begin with. The behaviour remains but the result is unhelpful, so breaking that connection between overeating and emotion at an unconscious level will enable you to move on to a more helpful relationship with food.

'Focused thinking' is best carried out in a 'light trance'. A trance is something you experience frequently – several times a day in fact. It's like daydreaming or that feeling you get between sleeping and waking. You might also have experienced it while driving and reaching your destination without really remembering the journey. These are all trance states and they allow your attention to be turned inwards and your unconscious mind to make changes free from the distraction of the outside world (and your internal voice). Of course, just like when you are daydreaming or driving, if something happens that requires your conscious awareness then you immediately become aware of the external world and can give it your full attention.

Before you embark on your own focused thinking or self-hypnosis, now is a good time to listen to the hypnotic recording that accompanies this part of the book. You can access this recording by going to http://www.inside-outweightloss.com and accessing the 'Client Area'. You need to enter the following password: WL125a

Action!   5: Focused Thinking

Practise focused thinking daily – it's a great way to relax and de-stress as well as to make changes at an unconscious level. Make sure you know all the steps before you start.

A   **Getting in the 'right state'**

Find a comfortable, quiet place where you can be undisturbed for half an hour.

Sit or lie down and focus your eyes on a spot above eye level. Stare at that spot intently noticing everything about it, notice also any sounds you can hear around you and notice how you feel. Breathe deeply and as you exhale, move your eyes downwards and just allow them to close.

With your eyes closed focus on your breathing, allowing it to become relaxed and even – and notice how relaxation can spread throughout your body until you feel calm, peaceful and comfortable.

Now allow your tongue to move from the top of your mouth so that it is relaxed and that internal voice starts to fade away so that all you notice is a quiet, peaceful place inside your head. Give that peaceful space a soothing colour and texture. Just allow the feeling to develop for a few minutes and enjoy it.

Congratulate yourself for taking control of your future wellbeing and for having all the resources you need to make change.

Practise this procedure a few times and then introduce some 'suggestions' by focusing your thinking. (Move on to part B)

Cont./

B   *Focusing your thinking*

Think about the situations where you overeat (refer back to your food-mood diary if necessary). Think about how you would like to act differently in those situations and imagine yourself doing it.

See yourself acting in the new, desired way and imagine what you would see, hear and feel.

Think about what you would say to yourself to describe what your new way of acting is e.g. "I consider what I want or need to eat from an objective point of view. I recognise when I am feeling an emotional need and find ways of tackling that without food". It's important that you phrase this in the positive tense.

Then think about what you could tell yourself to do in future when you encounter the situation in which you want to act differently e.g. "each time I feel angry and upset I will close my eyes, take several deep breaths and sort out what is making me feel that way and decide what I can do about it in a calm and rational way". Again this should be phrased positively.

So to summarise the steps for focused thinking:

1. *Think about the behaviour you want to change*
2. *Imagine yourself carrying out the new, desired behaviour*
3. *Put your new behaviour into words (in the present tense and stated in the positive)*
4. *Put into words your new strategy for responding to a trigger relating to your new behaviour (stated in the future tense and in the positive).*

Now put parts A and B together to give yourself a powerful tool to make changes at an unconscious level. Carry out regularly – every day if you can manage and add as many suggestions as you like (following the steps 1-4 for each one).

Taking stock

Well done for coming this far and completing 'On the Inside'. You have made lots of progress in gaining awareness of your eating habits and in making changes on a conscious and unconscious level to overcome compulsive and habitual eating.

Keep recording in your Food-Mood diary and spend some time now writing in your journal about how you have found your first steps towards changing your lifestyle forever. Keep practising your focused thinking as you move on to the next section – 'Taking Control'.

Taking Control

In this section: Re-setting your signalling system

A sensory experience

Who Says?

Now you are aware of the reasons why you overeat and are changing your eating behaviour away from being compulsive and habitual, you can move to a more natural and satisfying relationship with food.

By deciding when to eat in relation to your body's needs and making the experience of eating pleasurable, you will make your relationship with food a natural one, resulting in you feeling and looking your best. Learning to adapt your natural eating behaviours to different situations will mean you remain comfortably in control of when you eat.

Re-setting your signalling system

Periods of dieting, restricting calorie intake and alternating with cycles of overeating and abusing your body's natural hunger patterns will have interfered with your internal hunger signals. You may have gone for years without feeling physical hunger because you were too busy feeding your emotional hunger to allow yourself to become physically hungry. Or else you have starved yourself on diets and not fed your physical hunger – making your body think that it was being deprived of food, and so it held on to calories (energy) by way of storing fat – making you fat.

So you need to train yourself to eat only when you are physically hungry.

Action! 6: Deciding when to eat and when to stop

To begin with you might need to make a point of 'tuning in' to what's happening inside your body in order to recognise when you are really hungry. Do this every couple of hours and rate your hunger according to being:

- A. Not at all hungry
- B. Starting to feel the first twinges of hunger
- C. Hungry and would really like to eat now
- D. Ravenously hungry – would eat almost anything!

Physical hunger will progress through these stages (unlike emotional hunger which would hit you at C or D and make you want to grab something straight away).

You should eat when you are at C so you are ready to eat but not so hungry that you make an unhealthy choice. The more regularly you practise this the quicker it will become natural to recognise real hunger and you won't need to consciously 'tune in' after a little while.

Sometimes our bodies confuse the signals for thirst with the signals for hunger – especially if you are not used to reading the signals. Your 'hunger' might actually be thirst, so try drinking a glass of water regularly (about once an hour) so that your thirst doesn't interfere with your hunger signals.

Drinking plenty of water is also a great way to help your system start working naturally again – it helps to flush out toxins and get your metabolism working more efficiently.

Of course when you start eating – when you are hungry - you have to remember to stop eating when you have satisfied that hunger.

Cont/

35

Stop eating when you feel pleasantly full – not stuffed or uncomfortable. Learn to recognise the point at which you have physically had enough. Your body senses when you are full and sends you a signal to stop eating. You might have been so used to overriding this signal that you will have to train yourself to recognise it again.

If you eat slowly and focus on what you are eating you are more likely to recognise the signal that you are full. Notice how you feel as you eat, and at the point you start to enjoy your food less, stop eating. Give your brain time to let you know you are full by chewing slowly and paying attention to your meal.

It doesn't matter if you leave food on your plate – you are not wasting it – it would be a waste if you ate it all and felt bad afterwards. Try using a smaller plate and dishing up less – you can always have more if you are still hungry – but it removes the temptation to 'eat up'.

A sensory experience

You will have been used to eating because of the way it makes you feel rather than to enjoy the food for what it is – you would probably also have feelings of guilt afterwards coupled with the feelings that made you overeat in the first place. So now you are ready to move on to making when you eat a pleasurable experience – before, during and after.

When eating to satisfy an emotional need or habit you will not really have been noticing the taste of the food you were eating – just the feeling it gave you. Now you have broken that connection to emotion and habit you can focus on food as something pleasurable for its own sake. **Make a promise to yourself that you will only eat what you find really pleasurable to eat.**

If you have been dieting for years, having meal replacements or calorie-counting chances are you have compromised on the *taste* of your food. Pre-packaged ready meals and processed food are at best tasteless and mostly so laden with salt and artificial flavours that any natural tastes are completely camouflaged. To appreciate and enjoy food for what it is you need to *taste* it.

The artificial sweeteners and chemicals added to processed food are difficult for your body to break down and so the processes involved in breaking down fat and converting food to energy are diverted to deal with all the unnatural substances you are putting in your body. It follows then that artificial flavours and processed food make you fat – as well as unhealthy.

Case Study

Hazel, a mother of 3 had struggled with her weight for years and had reached the stage where she thought nothing would work for her. She lacked energy and was miserable. Just a few weeks after starting Inside-Out Weight Loss she had lost 11lbs and dropped 2 dress sizes.

She says *"it's completely changed my life; I eat what I want when I want and at long last have banished my 'love-hate' relationship with food – the guilt and self-loathing are in the past and that's where they will stay!"*

"With the program I completely eradicated my craving for chocolate, which was definitely a compulsive food for me, and now I haven't eaten any for 6 months"

Action! 7: Make Eating a Great Experience

STOP eating diet, low fat, reduced calorie, artificially sweetened and processed food

Take pride in preparing natural, good food for yourself and family/friends

Take time to enjoy and appreciate natural flavours – eat slowly and chew food well and deliberately

Eat what you truly find pleasurable – ask yourself before you eat –"do I want to eat this because I will enjoy the flavours, appearance and smell of it and appreciate every mouthful?"

Choose what you eat consciously (don't eat because you are bored or because it's 'time' to eat)

Focus on what you are eating – it's difficult to monitor whether you are full or not if you are not giving your meal your full attention

Enjoy developing an interest in different and new foods, combining flavours and creating meals

RESPECT your body and it's naturally balanced state with natural food and flavours. Your body will thank you by losing weight, filling you with energy, having clear skin and eyes, fighting off illness and achieving a general state of wellbeing.

Who Says?

Of course, you might still feel that despite changing your relationship with food – other peoples' relationships with food may still impact on you. As I said in the introduction, food – the offering and receiving of - is highly symbolic and you might feel pressure to eat in particular circumstances when you are not physically hungry or would choose not to eat what is offered. Your response in these situations is something you can learn to manage comfortably.

Situations such as visiting friends, family occasions, BBQs, dinner parties, dining out or meeting friends for coffee can be tricky if you are the sort of person who feels it's impolite to refuse an offer of dessert or cake or even an extra portion of potatoes. Restaurant portion sizes can be ridiculously huge, relatives might have baked you a cake especially, all your friends might be trying the new offerings at the coffee shop. All these things might present you with a dilemma – "do what others expect/want me to do" or "be true to myself and do what I really want".

In reality your perceived notion of offending others is probably unfounded. With the possible exception of your granny who has baked you a cake it's unlikely that anyone would insist on you eating something you don't want to! People will generally admire you for making changes to your lifestyle and compliment you on looking great. Others may try to encourage you to eat to make themselves feel better – they might be envious of your new confidence and respect for yourself. You might also be surprised by how many other people refuse offers of food with no trouble at all – or the many other people in the coffee shop quite happy to drink coffee on its own without an accompanying cake or muffin. Or the slim people at the dinner party who quietly leave food on their plate and politely refuse dessert without anyone noticing or objecting. You can be one of those people too. But, of course, if you are physically hungry, or really fancy a piece of cheesecake – then eat! Just be sure to follow what your body is telling you and stop when it's time to stop or you are no longer finding what you are eating pleasurable. You might start to find the portion sizes in restaurants off putting - it's perfectly acceptable to ask for a small plate and put what you think is a reasonable portion on that and leave the rest or ask them to take it away. You are paying for it – but that doesn't mean you have to eat it all. You are paying for a pleasurable experience so make sure it is!

Ensuring you are in a 'resourceful state' when you encounter any of these situations will make it easier for you to remain in control. If you feel that you are easily talked into things or still feel that 'expectation' towards you, then being able to pull on your resources of confidence and determination will be very useful.

Action! 8: Getting into a Resourceful State

Find a quiet spot and carry out the 'getting yourself in the right state' you use for focused thinking.

*Bring to mind a time when you felt full of **confidence and determination**, when you were able to do exactly as you wanted to do and had that feeling of strength and power. Take your time to come up with the best example of this you can find in your experience. If you can't think of a time, then you can think of someone who has those qualities, someone you admire, and think of how they would behave.*

Let the picture of that time (or other person) develop, noticing everything about it, how you looked, how you spoke, how others responded to you, how it felt. Now make the picture bigger and brighter, make the sounds clearer and louder. If you can make something better in the picture, do it until it is perfect.

*Now imagine stepping into that picture so you feel like you are actually there, seeing through your own eyes. Let yourself feel how it feels as you imagine the scene unfolding as if it is really happening – **your feelings of confidence and determination grow and grow, making you feel powerful and in control**. Now make a fist with your right hand and squeeze it tight as you let those feelings of confidence, determination and strength flood through you. Now release your fist, open your eyes for a moment and then close them again.*

Cont/

42

Now imagine a time and situation in the future where you might be faced with others' expectations to eat more than you want. Look at the picture as if it is a freeze frame from a movie. You can see yourself and others – perhaps you can see someone offering you a dessert or a dish full of chips, or maybe you are standing at the buffet table with friends as they tell you "you have to try the triple chocolate fudge cream cake" (or whatever else they are tempting you with!).

Imagine stepping right into that picture, just as the movie starts to play again, and this time you are actually in there seeing the scene with your own eyes. As the movie starts to play squeeze your right fist again and allow those feelings of confidence, determination and strength flood through you as you see yourself politely refusing offers and leaving what you don't want to eat. Feel how it feels to be in control and feel the admiration from others. Hear what you are saying and hear what others say to you – perhaps you are laughing at their insistence before they give in and accept your new way of being. Enjoy all those good feelings before you release your fist and open your eyes.

*Any time you feel you need to be in a more resourceful state you can **squeeze your fist and allow those feelings to come back.***

Taking stock

This section focused on using practical tools for increasing your control around eating – allowing you to respond to your body in a natural and respectful way. It encouraged you to make eating a good experience with good food and the resources to eat only when and what you really want.

You can now add new suggestions to your daily focused thinking so that becoming tuned into your body's naturally balanced state becomes unconscious.

Keep recording in your Food-Mood diary if you still find it useful and keep making entries in your journal to monitor your progress and success. Listen to the first recording again if you haven't already.

Making it Last - Forever

The previous 2 sections set the important groundwork for you to make significant and lasting changes to how you relate to food. Now we need to move onto creating a future that includes your new lifestyle and makes your changes 'sustainable, successful and satisfying'.

Creating your future
An important distinction to make is between setting goals and *creating a future.* Creating a future is an evolving process with successes and challenges along the way, and the future starts *right now.* Goals are something you set yourself to achieve at a specific point in the future – maybe weeks, months or years from now and once you achieve it - what then? Although goal setting may be useful in business or sport for example it doesn't leave room for all the personal triumphs and progress you make every day when creating a healthy, happy lifestyle – one that you will want to stay with you for the rest of your life. So, everyday imagine yourself creating a new slimmer, healthier you – just like a sculptor creating a masterpiece

work of art – bit by bit seeing it develop everyday and everyday being proud of what is created.

Two things you need to remember when thinking about creating your future are:

Make your future positive –think about the things you **do** want to happen and be, not what you don't want.

You have all the resources you need within you to make great changes and have the life you want, so you can start it happening now.

Spend some time writing in your journal about the future you want. What specifically you want your life to be like and how you see yourself making the journey. What the impact will be on others and on all the things you do now and the new things you will do in the future.

Action!   9: The future that's already there

Take some quiet time and close your eyes.

Imagine your life as a line with your past behind you and your future in front of you.

Now imagine you are floating above this line and can see your life below you.

See right into the future to the you that is celebrating your 90th birthday.

See the future you as having lived a life free from compulsive eating, free from self-doubt and criticism. The you that chose to change their life, leaving the old habits and unhealthy ways behind. See how healthy, happy and content you are.

Now float down into that future you so you feel you are right there, being you at that time. Take some time to see, hear and feel what is going on around you in this ideal future.

And now imagine that you are travelling back along your time line towards your present self. Stop each time you feel that you have something important to take from that moment - you don't necessarily need to know what it is, just pause for a moment and gather the resources from various points in your future life that help you in creating the future you want.

When you arrive back to your present self, you can imagine a connection to that future you – perhaps a ribbon, thread, rope or anything you like in any size, colour and texture – something that connects you to the future you and guides you along the way to the future that is already there.

Limiting beliefs

Sometimes even though you know what is the best way forward for you and you can comfortably see what your best future will look and be like – you still have beliefs about yourself that hold you back. If you have spent years yo-yo dieting and abusing your body with poor food you might have a pretty low opinion about yourself. Hopefully you stopped that inner voice criticising and being unhelpful with the action in the first section (if it's still there, go back and complete action 3 again until your internal voice is kind and encouraging). If you still believe that you don't have what it takes to make changes that will last forever and result in a new, slim, healthy you – now is the time to change that belief.

Action! 10: Change your Self-Limiting Beliefs

In your journal write down all the negative beliefs about yourself e.g. "I won't manage to sustain my weight loss because I always fail at everything eventually"

For each of your limiting beliefs imagine what it would be like if they were true and picture what your future would be like as a result.

Now imagine what that future would be like if the opposite of your belief was true e.g. "with the right approach and resources I make a success of everything I do". Step into that picture in your mind and experience what it feels like with that new belief.

Now write down at least 4 examples from your life that disprove your limiting beliefs and break them down into what you are actually pretty good at. Now ask yourself if that original belief is really true

Beliefs can change throughout life - there are plenty of things that you used to believe that you now know not to be true (Santa Claus, the Tooth Fairy, that your parents knew the answer to everything, or that anyone over the age of 30 was old). You can think of your old self-limiting beliefs as something you used to believe but now know not to be true.

Are you congruent?

Are all parts of you working together in creating your future or is there a conflict between different parts of you? Is there one part of you that is fully committed and excited about making changes and another part that is holding back for some reason? Do you often say "yes – but...." in answer to a question?

You have probably heard yourself saying at some point in your past "one part of me wants to ...... but another part doesn't". On some level both parts want the same thing for you but perhaps the reticent part feels it is protecting you from hurt/harm/disappointment and therefore keeping you safe. The motivated part of you also wants safety, security and success for you but creates this in a different way. Although the parts seem to be in conflict they are actually working towards the same outcome and just need help 'coming together'.

Addressing these parts of you as though they are separate will resolve any inner conflict that is stopping you being fully committed to the future you are creating for yourself. By moving these parts together the positive intentions will be focused in the same direction, to move you forward.

Action!   11: Resolving Inner Conflict

If you feel that there are parts of you in conflict, use this Action to resolve that conflict and integrate positive intentions.

Identify what it is that you want to move forward with and the reason for having difficulty. For example "I want to change the way I shop for and prepare food at home" **but** *"It will be too difficult to change my routine and fit in new ways of doing things – my life is too busy".*

Now, from your witness position, imagine these 2 different 'parts' of you as though you could fit them in each hand. Imagine what they would look like, sound like and what they might say to you. Imagine what feelings are connected to each part. Put your hands, palm up in front of you and imagine seeing and feeling those parts in your hands.

Now ask each part what positive intention they have for you. In the example, the first part might have as its intention to find new, healthier, natural food that you would use to create new, tasty, satisfying meals with. The other part wants to keep things simple for you, not add stress to your already busy life by changing routine.

Keep asking each part what that positive intention achieves for you until you reach a level of agreement i.e. the first part in the example wants a healthy life for you which will get you comfort and happiness. The other part of you wants familiarity and order which ultimately also gets you comfort and happiness (there might be just a few or many steps before you reach agreement on the ultimate positive intention of each part).

Cont/

51

From your witness position thank each part for its contribution and then ask them to move together to create a powerful combined part with the same ultimate positive intention for you.

As you do this allow your hands to move slowly together as you bring the parts together. When they meet, allow yourself to experience the feeling of the parts coming together in agreement and then pull your hands toward yourself to allow the new combined parts to integrate back into your body.

Note: You might find this easier to do in a light trance state so you can combine this Action with you focused thinking and 'being in a relaxed state'. Do this Action for all the different conflicting 'parts' of you and streamline your positive intentions.

Dealing with the set backs

Few journeys are completed without any obstacles or challenges along the way and it would be unreasonable to expect that your weight loss journey will be entirely smooth. Unless you live in a bubble cut off from everything, then life, relationships, work and the world in general will all have an impact on you.

There are times and situations that are demanding. Friends and family who expect different things from you and perhaps a job that takes a lot of your energy and time. Many things can cause you stress and stress can cause you to compound limiting beliefs (or make up new ones) and seek comfort by feeding your emotions.

Dealing with stress quickly and effectively will release you from the feeling that you need to 'cover it up' or manage it with destructive behaviour. Often after you have managed your stress in a situation you can have more clarity of thought and determine what the issue really is – rather than allowing stress to 'blow things out of proportion' or for you to make up potentially catastrophic outcomes in your head that (most probably) will never happen.

Action! 12: Managing Stress Quickly and Easily

Practise this action a few times so that when you next encounter a situation that you find stressful and could potentially send you off track you know what to do to manage it.

Find a quiet spot (it doesn't have to be anywhere special just a place where you can be alone for a few minutes). If possible sit down but you can do this standing up if necessary. Notice what is around you, what you can see, hear and feel and then close your eyes and notice what you can hear and feel. Allow your breathing to become even (don't breath too deeply but just let it settle).

Notice any tenseness in your body and let it relax – starting from your head and neck (allow your tongue to go loose in your mouth), down your arms and body and then your legs, finishing with your feet and toes. Let all the tension go.

As your breathing becomes even, start breathing from your diaphragm (so you can feel your stomach expand as you breath in) and as you do so, keep your mind clear, let any thoughts go.

Imagine your stress or anxiety as a cloud or puff of smoke leaving your body and blowing away on the wind as you exhale.

As you inhale, imagine that a coloured or bright light spreads throughout your body –filling you up with a sense of calm and control, making you peaceful and strong, poised and resourceful.

Keep allowing that light to spread through you giving you all you need to deal with those stressful situations and the old anxious feelings to disappear in the breeze.

You are creating a new future and if you feel that you have let yourself down or gone off track at any point, it's just part of the journey. An obstacle on the road doesn't mean you stop and go back to the beginning, you find a way around it, you learn to deal with other similar obstacles and move on. Use the tools and techniques you have already learnt to deal with challenges and become stronger and more confident each time.

Action!   13: Focused Thinking

You can now add your connection to your future self to your focused thinking. Imagine the future you at the furthest point in the future having created a sustainable, satisfying and successful lifestyle. Then see yourself at various stages back from the future until now. Choose the image of you that you like the best – maybe it is you just a few months from now looking great, happy and full of vitality - or perhaps an older you settled and content with your life.

Make that image big, bright, colourful and vivid. You can bring this image to mind any time to remind you of what you are creating and it can pull you towards your future.

Keep suggesting to yourself the beliefs you now have in yourself and for your future

Finally, congratulate yourself for making such amazing changes!

Taking stock
You have come a long way since starting Inside-Out
Weight loss:

You have:

- Become aware of your relationship with food, broken the emotional connection to food and developed new strategies to eliminate habitual eating.
- Changed that internal voice from critical and abusive to kind and encouraging.
- Learned to focus your thinking and use it regularly, along with the recording to make changes at an unconscious level.
- Re-set your internal signalling system so you only eat when you are physically hungry and stop when you are full.
- Started to respect your naturally balanced state so that you taste and appreciate real food and eat only what you find truly pleasurable to eat.
- Learned to deal with the expectations of others and call upon a resourceful state.
- Developed a clear idea of what you want your future to be and how to create it.
- Dealt with limiting beliefs and inner conflict and have an effective strategy for managing stress.

Case Study

Yvonne 'yo-yo' dieted for years and felt her eating habits were out of control. After just one week using the Inside-Out program she noticed a huge difference in her relationship with food and her whole attitude towards eating became more relaxed without thinking or worrying about it. She was amazed at how easily the weight came off.

She says *"over the past couple of months my weight has reduced drastically without me having to starve myself or eat unappealing diet foods. I don't feel at all like I am dieting and actually hardly ever consciously think about food at all – a huge change for me!"*

"I have dropped 2 dress sizes with the program already and get much more pleasure from seeing my clothes get looser and looser than I do from tucking into yet another chocolate bar"

Acknowledging and changing your relationship with food from the inside-out = sustainable, successful and satisfying weight loss

The next two Parts build on your progress so far and give you additional guidance for wellbeing and healthy weight loss, including how to deal with unhelpful food cravings and how to build motivation to exercise.

Part Two

Choices

Part 2 is about giving you additional tools and knowledge so you can make choices to support your new, healthier relationship with food.

By completing Part 1 you will have broken the cycle of compulsive and habitual eating and will have new feelings of control around food. You are able to choose what you really want to eat when you are physically hungry and stop when you are full.

Now you can build on your new positive relationship with food and maximise the nutritional benefit for wellbeing – helping you to feel and look great.   This section is about giving you simple nutritional information to guide you towards making healthy choices and the means to make those preferences unconscious. That way, healthy eating will become a part of your normal day-to-day lifestyle.

Be sure to carry out the Actions, incorporate new suggestions into your focused thinking and listen to the accompanying recording. As before, the recording can be found at www.inside-outweightloss.com from the Client Area using password WL125a .

A Balanced Outlook

Throughout Inside-Out Weight Loss I refer to respecting your body's naturally balanced state. Being able to maintain this naturally balanced state requires us to give ourselves what we need mentally and physically and eliminate factors that upset the balance.

In Part 1 you have already re-set your emotional balance, learnt to recalibrate and respond to your physical signals and developed effective ways to deal with external factors that impact on your internal balance.

You will probably be aware of the fact that eating or lacking certain types of food can also upset your internal balance. Sometimes the physical symptoms of imbalance can be quite dramatic (pain, bloating, skin breakouts etc.), but other symptoms of imbalance can manifest as irritability, tiredness, low mood or energy and a general negative impact on wellbeing.

Some of the more extreme diets that restrict food groups or focus on only particular types of food have such dramatic physical and emotional side effects that it is no wonder that hardly anyone can endure them for long.

My advice is to respect your body's naturally balanced state – how it was designed to be- and eat a balanced range of foods from all of the food groups. Eating a broad range of foods will maximise your nutritional intake and therefore maximise the likelihood that you will get all the recommended levels of vitamins, minerals and macro nutrients (fats, carbohydrates and protein).

Proportionally thinking

Eating a balanced range of foods means balancing your intake in relation to what *your body needs to stay healthy.* The British FSA (Food Standards Agency) and American USDA (United States Department of Agriculture) both recommend a diet high in vegetables and fruits (approx. one third of your intake) and starchy whole grain food (another third of your intake). The remaining proportion of your food intake is ideally split between protein and dairy foods.

Eating healthily can be very simple indeed – just remember to keep it simple! All of our food falls within 5 major food groups: vegetables, fruits, starchy foods (including grains), non-dairy protein and milk/dairy products. My 3 golden rules for keeping healthy eating simple are:

1. Think in thirds: one third vegetables and fruits, another third starchy foods/grains and the remaining third protein and dairy products
2. Remember that not all foods are equal within the food groups (see fats, carbs and protein on the next page)
3. Try to consume food in its most nutritionally dense form i.e. without added salt, fats, sugars or processing (including artificial sweetening, flavouring and preserving)

More or Less

There are lots of myths around eating *fats, carbs and protein* and a lot of the 'miracle diets' are based on these myths. The **truth** is that eliminating entire macro-nutrients (fats, carbs and protein) from your diet can result in severe malnutrition and life threatening medical disorders.

Fats (and oils) are necessary for many processes in your body such as forming cell membranes, for nerve and brain function and in hormone formation. Fat is also necessary so your body can process vitamins A, E, D and K —essential for healthy skin, hair, eye sight, bones, blood and as anti-oxidants. However, not all fats are equal!

In *general* fats from animal meat and products (including most full fat milk products and cheese) is high in saturated fat that can be damaging to health if you have a lot of it. Fats in processed food such as pastries, cakes, cookies, biscuits etc. can be 'trans-fats' which are also damaging to your health if you consume a lot. On the other hand, fats found in oily fish, nuts, plant oils and seeds are beneficial to health (especially the omega 3 and 6 oils), and you can get all the necessary dietary fats requirements from them.

Carbohydrates (carbs) are the main source of energy in the body and come in many forms. If you deliberately restrict carbohydrates in your diet, your body eventually starts to use protein for energy and literally starts to eat your muscles – this is very dangerous and could result in a heart attack and death. The absorption and distribution of carbs around the body impacts on blood sugar levels giving you that boost and slump in energy and the cravings for certain foods. The carbohydrates that are converted to blood sugar more slowly to give a more stable source of energy are preferable to the 'quick fix' carbs which result in a 'spike' in energy followed by a dramatic slump.

The Glycaemic Index (GI) is how carbohydrates are classified in terms of how quickly they are processed and absorbed by the body. Foods that have a low GI contribute to more stable blood sugar levels (therefore minimising the spikes and slumps) and those with a high GI are digested more quickly, giving a quick energy boost but a rapid decrease in blood sugar shortly afterwards. Low GI foods make you feel full for longer and high GI foods will result in you feeling hungry again soon after eating.

A lot of the foods we buy in supermarkets have their GI rating indicated on the packaging, so it's good to look for low GI foods. These include new potatoes, oats, pulses, wheat pasta, sweet potato, apples and oranges. High GI foods include white and whole meal bread, crackers, chips, cakes, biscuits and sweets. It's a good idea to include a low GI food with every meal, as this will have an overall stabilising impact on your blood sugar levels.

Protein is essential to build cells and tissue and for many basic functions. If you don't get enough protein in your diet (which is rare unless a very low carbohydrate diet results in protein deficiency), your body starts to digest the protein present in your muscles and other tissues. Too much protein intake will put a strain on your kidneys and if a significant amount of that excess protein comes from meat, it may contain a high level of saturated fat that could put you at risk of heart disease. Some low/no carb diets recommend a diet consisting mainly of protein – this is not healthy. Good sources of protein are – eggs, lean meat, poultry, soya beans, nuts, seeds and pulses. Red meat is also a good source of protein but can contain high levels of saturated fat so other sources of protein are preferable.

Simple Steps
Following these guidelines and the following simple steps will help stabilise your blood sugar and metabolism and contribute to a healthy, nutrition rich food intake aiding weight loss. You could copy out these steps and keep them in your kitchen to remind you. A down-loadable version of the Simple Steps is also available at www.inside-outweightloss.com/resources-and-downloads.

Action!   14: Simple steps for healthy eating

- Respect your body's naturally balanced state
- Eat a wide range of foods to maximise nutritional benefit
- Remember all the food groups are essential to good health
- Eat foods in their nutritionally dense form i.e. limit added salt, sugar, fats, flavourings and preservatives
- Avoid processed foods which strip the nutritional value from the ingredients
- Eat organic when you can
- Have vegetables and starchy foods as the main components of your meals
- Include 'good' fats/oils in your meals to provide a source of essential fatty acids and omega 3 and 6
- Choose low GI (slow release) carbohydrates and include them as a part of every meal
- Choose sources of protein that are free from saturated fat
- Drink plenty of water to aid digestion and cleanse your system
- Eat breakfast – it 'jump starts' your metabolism (your body's mechanism for turning food into energy) after it has slowed down overnight
- Avoid eating late at night when your metabolism naturally slows down to conserve energy for when you sleep
- Cook food appropriately – eat veg and fruit raw as much as possible to retain its natural state and nutritional value
- Dispose of your microwave! Microwaving food destroys its nutrients. You will also be less tempted to have 'ready-meals' (which are highly processed, high in fat, sugar and salt and low in nutritional value) if you can't blast it in the microwave.
- Remember to eat when you are reasonably hungry not when you think you 'should', and stop when you are full

Cravings

No matter how good our intentions and well balanced our diets are we all still have the occasional craving for something that we would prefer to be able to resist. Maybe it is chocolate, cake or chips –something you think is sabotaging your progress and intentions to sustain a healthy, nutrition rich lifestyle. Your body is shouting out for it, but your mind is saying 'no'. You can help your mind to control your cravings and convince your body it doesn't need it with a simple and very effective technique. Read the next Action carefully before you carry it out.

Action!   15: Banish Your Cravings

Decide on the food that you often have a craving for and want to eliminate from your diet (it's important that this is something that you would be happy not to want to eat ever again).

Close your eyes and bring to mind what that food looks like, what it smells like what it tastes like, the texture of it in your mouth and the sensation you get when you chew and swallow it.   Imagine eating a huge portion of it right now – experiencing all the sensations that go with it.

Open your eyes and think of something that you would really hate to eat – something that is disgusting to you – like dirt from the ground, the scum that lurks in the drains, a ball of dog hair or the contents of your vacuum cleaner. Or perhaps there is food that you find truly disgusting – one that you just can't stomach. Close your eyes and bring that to mind now – imagine its appearance, texture and smell – see it on a plate in front of you, as if it were really there.

Now, keeping your eyes closed, imagine a combination of the food you crave and the food or thing you find disgusting. Imagine them mixing together – combining all the smells, textures and tastes. Imagine a huge plate of the mixture in front of you – the smell wafting all around you. See that mixture coming towards you now and imagine the taste as you put it in your mouth.

Make a chewing motion with your mouth as you experience the texture of that disgusting mixture in your mouth, as you can taste the disgusting taste and experience the disgusting smell as you try to swallow it. Perhaps you gag as it reaches your throat and you think about swallowing it.....

Cont/

Now every time you think of the food you used to crave you can imagine the same sensations and tastes and find the thought of it truly disgusting!

(Another tip that people find useful is to go and clean your teeth when you are craving something – you will be surprised how having clean teeth and fresh, minty breath can stop that craving.)

Focused Thinking

You can add new suggestions to your focused thinking in the same way you did in Part 1. These suggestions can help you to make healthy choices when you are shopping, eating out, preparing meals at home and selecting snacks.

For example:
"each time I shop for food at the supermarket I visit the fruit and veg aisles first and enjoy the variety and choice of bright, vibrant, nutrition rich fruit and vegetables" – "I make most of my purchases single ingredient items (i.e. not pre-prepared packaged food- or foods with added ingredients) that I can use to prepare healthy meals"

"I ignore the aisles in the supermarket that are packed full of biscuits, crisps, sugary drinks and processed foods – knowing that in doing so I am respecting my body and its naturally balanced state"

"When I eat out, I make healthy choices from the menu. I choose nutrient dense meals to appreciate natural flavours and good quality food"

"I prepare nutritious food at home for myself and my family. I enjoy preparing a wide variety of healthy ingredients – combining flavours, aromas, colours and textures. I am doing the best for myself and my family by maximising the nutrition in the meals I prepare."

The recording
Listen to the recording that accompanies this section regularly (from the Client Area of www.inside-outweightloss.com password WL125a). It supports what you have learnt and helps to make changes at an unconscious level to make them part of your normal day-to-day lifestyle.

Taking stock
Part 2 focused on developing a healthy approach to what you eat in order to make your choices high in nutrition. Good nutrition is vital to staying healthy, looking good and maintaining energy levels. Following the steps, carrying out the actions, incorporating suggestions into your focused thinking and listening to the recording will result in an enhanced, healthy relationship with food that supports your weight loss outcomes.

You can now move onto the third and final part, which will support you to incorporate activity into your lifestyle.

Part Three

Integrating Activity

Part 3 is all about being active. Being active is not about sweating for hours at the gym or running for miles on the streets, or even enduring an exuberant aerobics session – unless of course that is what you enjoy doing.   Being active is about increasing your heart rate enough to have a positive impact on weight loss and your health.

Again, this part has Activities to complete and an accompanying recording – accessed from the website as before. Listen to the recording regularly and keep carrying out your own focused thinking to embed changes at an unconscious level.

Activity for weight loss

Let's look back to the original and widely accepted formula for losing weight:

Energy in (i.e. calories from food and drink) < Energy out

You have resolved issues impacting on your relationship with food and reduced 'energy in' by eliminating compulsive and habitual eating and by 're-programming' your internal signals. By increasing your 'energy out' you can further increase the differential, and lose weight even faster.

Most people would agree that *burning* extra energy through being active is a lot less noticeable than *reducing* energy-in by the same amount. For instance, a half hours brisk walk could use up the same amount of energy as you take in with half of your dinner-time meal. Walking for half an hour won't result in you feeling hungry, but only eating half of your meal probably will. Therefore, being more active is a very effective way to lose weight and also has many positive impacts on your fitness levels, health and wellbeing.

Your metabolism is your body's mechanism for turning food into energy. Activity levels impact on how efficiently your metabolism works – and keeping active speeds up the process not only during periods of activity but for many hours afterwards too. Increased metabolism means you convert food to energy more effectively and therefore lose weight quicker. So by being active everyday you can boost your metabolism and keep it working at an optimal level on a continuous basis.

Activity for wellbeing

Being over-weight puts you at a greater risk of high blood pressure, heart disease, stroke, diabetes and some cancers. Being overweight also increases the likelihood of bone and joint pain and inactivity can put you at higher risk of osteoporosis. Increased, regular activity can prevent or significantly reduce the impact of these disorders.

Increased, regular activity has also been proven to have a positive impact on anxiety and stress related disorders and has a beneficial effect on depressive conditions – without the side effects of medication.

Increasing activity releases endorphins in your brain that make you feel good and feel less stressed and anxious. Before, you may have got this 'fix' from overeating – but now you have broken that connection – a much better way to achieve that natural high is through increased activity.

For general wellbeing, keeping active on a regular basis will make you feel and look good, keep you mobile and strong as you get older, help with joint pain, improve circulation, help you sleep better and positively influence a wide range of health issues.

You should consult your doctor if you have any concerns about increasing your activity levels.

What is 'Being Active?'

Becoming more active is easy. Anything that increases your heart rate, gets you breathing harder and makes you warm is aerobic activity. Aerobic activity gets your heart and muscles working harder and that causes you to use up more energy and therefore lose weight. It stimulates your metabolism to generate more energy for your muscles to work and gets it working more efficiently.

You might have noticed your heart rate increasing when you do things like housework, gardening, climbing the stairs, carrying shopping bags or walking the dog. This is all activity and it is all good for weight loss and wellbeing. Do a bit more of it and feel and see the benefits. It doesn't have to be called exercise to be good for you! Walking is one of the best and easiest ways of keeping active and it's simple to fit in to your routine. You can start off walking a bit more each day – perhaps walking to the shops instead of taking the car, or walking the kids to school – and then increase the activity level of your walking routine by extending your route or varying the terrain.

Being active also means getting 'involved'. Getting fit and active is fun and you can combine it with meeting new people and doing something different and rewarding. Perhaps participating in a charity walk, volunteering at a youth group, organising events, or joining a golf club for example – these give you the opportunity to get involved with other people and activities and get fit at the same time.

Maximising the power

However you choose to be more active, you can start with as little or as much as you want and build up to a level of activity that supports your weight loss approach and enhances your wellbeing. Sometimes however you might allow yourself to let feelings of lethargy (a general feeling of listlessness or dis-inclination to do anything) prevent you from being more active and find it difficult to break out of the lethargy cycle. i.e. you feel lacking in energy so you don't bother to do anything active, you feel down about being inactive and so feel less likely to do anything about it, compounding your low energy levels and feelings of lethargy. You can easily break out of this cycle and feel the benefits of being more active -boosting your energy and mood. Carry out the following Action to set you off on a more active lifestyle and use it anytime you have feelings of lethargy creeping up on you.

Action: 16: Maximise the Power
                   - Limit the Lethargy

Think of the way you act when you have thought about exercising but feel disinclined to get going – maybe you can even visualise what you look or act like when you feel this way. What picture do you get in your head at the moment you decide you can't be bothered to exercise? (Maybe you imagine yourself sweaty and uncomfortable or panting with exhaustion for example) Create that picture in your mind, and imagine being at that moment with that thought and picture in your head.

Give yourself a shake, and think of someone that is motivated and determined to succeed in all areas of their life (you don't need to know them personally), what would you act like if you had those qualities? Bring a picture to mind of you being motivated and determined to bring yourself to better health and perfect wellbeing. See this image as a picture – make any changes you need to the picture to make it something that is completely acceptable in your life. Give yourself a little shake again.

Now close your eyes and imagine a computer screen in front of you with the old picture (the one of you with the old, undesired behaviour) filling the screen. Make the picture big and bright. Feel like you are stepping into the old you so that you are actually there looking out from your own eyes. In the bottom left hand corner of the screen imagine the new picture of the motivated you as a small, dark picture, where you can see yourself in the picture.

Cont/

Very quickly, have the 2 images swap places so the new, motivated you fills the screen as a big, bright image – and the old image minimises to the small, dark image in the corner – imagine a 'whooshing' noise as they swap places.

Allow the screen to go blank and open your eyes.

Repeat the fast swapping process many times (up to 10 or 12 times) – clearing the screen and opening your eyes between each time. This should be done super fast. Keep going until you cannot easily bring the old image to mind.

After several times of doing this you will find that it is difficult to bring the old image back up and you will feel like you are fully inside the new image of yourself – being motivated and determined to exercise.

Now close your eyes again and think of a situation where it is an ideal time for you to go and exercise. How do you feel now? If you are feeling motivated and determined – let the feeling grow and the image to get brighter and more appealing – and then squeeze your left hand into a fist as you keep the feeling going. Release your fist and open your eyes. (If you are not feeling motivated and determined in this situation go back and repeat the picture swapping exercise, but think carefully about the 'old you' image – make sure it is something you can fully associate with (something real) – at the point where you would decide NOT to go ahead and exercise).

You will now find that in the future where you experience the decision making point where you decide whether to exercise or not – instead of that trigger evoking feelings of lethargy – you will feel motivated to exercise. You can maximise this power and keep it going by squeezing your left hand into a fist!

Absorbing activity

The key to fitting additional activity into your life is to make it varied, interesting, enjoyable and convenient. A lot of people claim to not have the time or opportunity to exercise or be more active – perhaps because they work full time or have small children or other commitments. The truth is that **everyone** can be more active if they find appropriate ways to do it.

Both the UK Chief Medical Officer and the US Department of Health recommend 150 minutes of moderate intensity aerobic exercise every week for adults in order to improve health. This is 30 minutes a day spread over 5 days or a little more than 21 minutes a day over 7 days. Of course if you do more, you will increase your energy-out to energy-in differential and lose weight more quickly. Exercising in small 'chunks' is just as effective as longer sessions, so fitting in two 10 minute brisk walks or a play in the park with the kids could be more than an adequate amount of extra activity for one day for example.

If you work full time, you could easily find time to walk at lunch time or on the way to or from work. Perhaps get on or off the bus a couple of stops away from your usual or park further away from the office, or use the stairs more. Those short bursts of activity add up and you will soon see the benefit.

If you are at home with children – use their natural pre-disposition to be active to your advantage and start walking more with them – noticing all the new things you see or experience. Play in the park, invest in a bike with a child seat or trailer, go swimming, play football - the only limit to the activity and fun is your own and your kids' imaginations – and they will love it.

Look for and notice opportunities throughout your day to add to your activity levels and clock up those energy expending minutes. Welcome the opportunities as a resource to bring you closer and closer to your weight loss and fitness outcomes and feel good about yourself for taking them.

If you want to be more formal about your activity times – make appointments with yourself and don't break them. Commit by writing your appointments to exercise in your diary – like you would with an arrangement to meet another person, and stick to it.

Most of all – make activity an **integral part of your life**. Enjoy being an active person. If you find yourself slumped in front of the TV – get up and move around, do something else – make a pact with yourself not to be immobile for long periods of time (unless of course you are sleeping!). Small bursts of activity add up and **do you good**.

Focused thinking

You can add suggestions to your focused thinking to build on your motivation and determination to be active and promote your physical wellbeing. This will support the changes you have already made and re-enforce them at an unconscious level.

For example:

"I find opportunities throughout my day to be active and enjoy the feeling of exercising my body and the benefits that brings"

"Whenever I have been inactive for a period of time I have the urge to get up, move around, and get my heart beating faster and blood pumping to my muscles"

"I make a determined effort to walk more throughout the day – finding ways to build walking into my normal routine"

"I enjoy the health benefits that being active brings. I feel more energetic and full of life. I like the way that my body becomes more toned and slim and notice the admiring glances I get from other people"

The recording

Listen regularly to the recording that accompanies this part. It supports what you have learnt and helps to make changes at an unconscious level to make them part of your normal day-to-day lifestyle.

Taking stock

Part 3 focused on promoting and supporting your weight loss by increasing your activity levels. It gave you information and motivational techniques to make exercise and activity an integral part of your life. By incorporating healthy eating and exercise into your lifestyle along with the changes you have made to your relationship with food, you are giving yourself what you need to stay slim and healthy.

Congratulations on completing Inside-Out Weight Loss and I sincerely hope that you continue to benefit from the freedom to live your life in your own, naturally balanced state.

www.inside-outweightloss.com gives you additional support in your weight loss outcomes and creating your future. Please also feel free to contact me using the contact details on the website if you would like further information regarding weight loss, NLP or Hypnotherapy.

Appendix

NLP and Hypnotherapy for Weight Loss

NLP is short for Neuro-Linguistic Programming and looks at our subjective experiences and the structure and processes of our thinking and behaviour. Through various techniques and interventions NLP can help change the patterns of thought that lead to unhelpful behaviour. NLP for weight loss is particularly effective because most of our eating behaviours and habits are as a result of many different experiences, influences and deep-seated conditioning. Tackling those behaviours at a fundamental level through NLP replaces unhelpful patterns with positive, healthy ones.

Hypnotherapy has been used for centuries as a way of effecting change at an unconscious level – and therefore bypassing conscious barriers and challenges that make it difficult to break habits or overcome past trauma. Hypnosis or 'trance' is a completely natural state that you enter into spontaneously several times a day. When day dreaming for example or that common 'driving trance' where you arrive at your destination without remembering the journey because you were so absorbed in your own thoughts. Contrary to some perceptions you are not 'asleep' in hypnosis but in an altered state of awareness that allows you to focus internally and accept suggestions for change. You will only accept suggestions that are congruent with your values and your desire to change.

Hypnotherapy for weight loss is especially effective because compulsive eating is as a result of unconscious behaviour – usually in connection to seeking comfort, solace or diversion. Hypnotherapy can break the connection and allow the unconscious mind to provide the same positive intention with another, more helpful behaviour.

Also from MX Publishing

Seeing Spells Achieving

The UK's leading guide for parents and teacher for children with learning difficulties such as Dyslexia, ADD and ADHD.

Bridges To Success

When you know something works you have to teach others. Learn how to transform learning difficulties into successful learning differences, enabling youngsters and adults alike to succeed. Bridges to Success offers visually talented yet challenged individuals a completely new perspective, empowering them to change themselves and the system around them.

The Engaging NLP Series

A series of practical guides applying NLP to everyday life. NLP for Children, NLP for Parents, NLP for Teachers and more specific guides such as NLP Back To Work for mothers returning to work after having children.

CPSIA information can be obtained at www.ICGtesting.com
Printed in the USA
LVOW10s1929111214

418361LV00030B/1262/P